He Has UP Syndrome Not DOWN Syndrome

Caroline Brandt

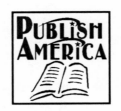

PublishAmerica
Baltimore

First printing

ISBN: 1-4137-6041-4
PUBLISHED BY PUBLISHAMERICA, LLLP
www.publishamerica.com
Baltimore

Printed in the United States of America

With love and admiration, I dedicate this book to my daughter Misty for being a dedicated mother and wife, a beautiful person and an inspiration to all those who know her. Thank you from the bottom of my heart for all of your encouragement and help with this book. Hopefully others with Down syndrome children will see what we see, that these people are wonderful, happy, upbeat people.

CHAPTER ONE

HE CAME TO US ON October 19, 2000, at noon. Riley Joe Hoofman weighed in at 5 lbs. 12 oz. and I was there for the birth. After he had been cleaned up and swaddled and Mom and Dad had held him, it was my turn. He was so light; he had good color and all the fingers and toes were counted. He opened his eyes for a minute and his left eye seemed to wander a bit. That could easily be fixed, I thought. He was gorgeous. Riley was my second grandson and Misty's second child. I was an ecstatic grandmother. They called me Momo.

Misty and Brent were very excited over the birth of their first child together. They each had a son by a previous marriage. Brent's son Zachary was four and Misty's son Cheyenne was eight. They knew their marriage and their child would be great. They were a happy, healthy young couple.

Misty was my oldest daughter. She was twenty-three and Brent, her second husband, was twenty-six. They had been married for a year. Misty had been through a lot in her short life. She married at fifteen and had her first son at sixteen. At that point, she was not my favorite child. She had been rebellious and disrespectful since her dad and I had divorced.

Her dad had been a functional alcoholic that I was married to for almost sixteen years. When we divorced, he became belligerent with me, calling and threatening me, my friends and my family. Then he began to confide in Misty, like she was an adult, at age fourteen. He tried to alienate Misty and I at that point, telling her things that should not be shared with a fourteen-year-old girl. He and she were pretty close; however, Misty began to realize that her father was sick.

Then her father died in a single vehicle accident in January 1997 as he was driving home drunk, from seeing his third wife, who he was separated from. He was only forty-two years old and the truck caught fire after he crashed into a telephone pole.

Misty raised Cheyenne by herself for the first two years while her first husband, Jeremy, went through drug rehab in Houston, Texas. After the rehab, they lived together as husband and wife for almost two years. But since then he had remarried and it was during this stressful time (of her dad's death) that Jeremy, her now ex-husband, managed to obtain primary custody of their son, Cheyenne.

Now, back to that day. It was about five p.m. and Cheyenne was brought to the hospital by his dad and step-mom, Karen, to see his new brother and his mom. He was very excited and was looking forward to having another brother. We all visited for a while and were talking and laughing. Everyone had finally reached a point where it was okay to be around each other. Jeremy and Karen finally left to go home, and Brent was going to take Cheyenne home later that evening.

Then the doctor came to the room and wanted everyone to leave for a few minutes. I thought he was going to examine Misty for some reason, so I left cheerfully.

After about twenty minutes I was asked to come in the room. Misty was crying and Brent was red-eyed. I asked, "What? What is wrong?" I was really nervous.

Misty said, "Mom, sit down....Riley has Down syndrome." She was crying.

I said, "No way, how can they know that...he looks fine to me, no way." Deep down, I wondered about the eye and how it seemed to wander, and then I thought, *No way, that just cannot be.*

She said, "They ran some physical tests and they are running several blood tests that will tell us for sure, but they take several weeks. However, the doctor says he has low muscle tone, his neck is shorter than what is normal, his fingers are short and stubby, and he has the almond eyes. Also, there might be another problem...his oxygen levels in his blood are low and they do not know why yet. They are running more tests to find out. So, they are going to be putting him in the neonatal intensive care unit to put him on oxygen for his breathing."

I thought, *Oh my dear Lord, this cannot be happening, not to us, no way. They are young and healthy, and this is just a bad dream. Besides that, what is low muscle tone, what does that mean? What does it matter if he has a short neck? I like cute stubby fingers. But I have to keep calm, keep this to myself.*

"Misty, Brent, it will be okay," I said. "They are wrong…you will see. No matter what happens, it will be fine, you will see." I wondered if they believed me, because I did not believe a word I said.

"Look, Mom, can you take Cheyenne back to his dad's? I don't want him to see us this upset," Misty asked.

"I guess so. That's going to be kind of hard for me to do because I am so upset, but I will. I just have to compose myself."

Heather, my youngest daughter, had walked into the room. Heather was nineteen years old, attending college and living in Denton, Texas. Denton is about thirty miles north of Fort Worth and Dallas. She was very supportive, telling Misty and Brent it would all work out, to try and stay calm, that Riley would be a blessing.

She had been around a severely disabled child for a couple years with her high school boyfriend's brother, Jordan. She had become very attached to him over the two years they had dated, and then she and Josh had broken up before they both went off to college. Heather was being very compassionate about Riley's suspected condition.

I kissed them both and left, holding back the hysteria. I had to. I needed to take Cheyenne home and not upset him, and it was about a twenty-minute drive.

Cheyenne and I talked the whole way about his new little brother and how much fun it would be to have someone to play with. We talked about school and how he liked his teacher and his classmates. He was very talkative and I was so glad. I did not want him to see how I was really feeling.

We got to his dad's house and Karen came out with red eyes. Misty had called her to let her know what was going on so that they could find a way to break it to Cheyenne. I kissed Cheyenne goodbye and looked at Karen and said, "I got to go. I am sorry, I can't talk about this yet."

As I was driving down Saginaw Boulevard in Saginaw, Texas, a little suburb of Fort Worth, I was overcome with emotion and I pulled over to the side of the road. I called Lisa, my business partner and best friend, on my cell phone. I was hysterical crying, and I couldn't stop. She could barely understand what I was saying. She was very comforting, telling me it would be all right, and we would figure it out, not to worry. Somehow she managed to calm me down enough that I could think.

Then I called Bob, my husband, and told him. He could not believe it. He told me to calm down and come home. I got home fifteen minutes later and just collapsed in his arms sobbing. It was about seven in the evening when I got there. After I calmed down, I told Bob I had to go back to the hospital to be with Misty and Brent. It was just too much to handle alone. He was very supportive and told me to do whatever I felt I needed to do. So I drove back over to the hospital.

When I got there, they were a little calmer and Misty told me, "Brent and I talked about it and prayed about it a lot already. We will handle this. We will take care of him and do whatever we have to do. He is our son. God sent him to us and we will do whatever may be necessary. The only thing that really worries me, Mama, is that people won't love him. They won't have anything to do with him because he is different."

I couldn't believe she had even said that. "No way, Misty. He will be loved no matter what. I promise you," I said, trying to hold back the tears.

A few minutes later the nurse brought Riley in the room. We took turns holding our Riley Joe and praying under our breath that the doctors were wrong. Then Lisa, my best friend and the godmother, came in the door with Nancy, her friend. *Oh, thank God,* I thought. *What a comfort...how great...driving over from Dallas to make sure we are okay.*

The nurse came in to get Riley and take him back to the nursery. They were becoming very concerned about his condition and wanted to monitor him more closely.

Everyone talked and visited and laughed, trying to pretend it was not real. Soon we figured that we had stayed as long as we could and decided to leave.

"Misty," I said, "I will be back in the morning. Try to get some rest and quit worrying."

The next morning came very quickly. I got up at six and was on my way by seven in the morning. I rushed as fast as I could to get to the hospital. I was so nervous that something might go wrong. My heart was just racing while I was driving.

Misty and Brent were up and they explained to me that the doctors thought there might be a problem with his heart. The pediatric cardiologist told them that Riley had two holes in his heart. This was a common defect in Down's babies and it was not necessarily as serious as it sounded. They were going to monitor him and run more tests. We would only be able to see Riley in the NICU, but they would keep us informed.

"You can go to see him, Mom, but not everyone will be able to go to NICU to see him. They are putting him under a bilirubin light for jaundice, and they are giving him oxygen and will be monitoring all of his vitals. It does not look good."

"Well, let's just stay calm and let them do their jobs and figure out what is going on," I said.

"Mom, he might not be able to go home with me when they discharge me," Misty cried. She was just a bundle of nerves.

"Okay," I said, "let's just wait and see how it goes."

We were hugging each other and just watching each other's facial expressions when…

All of a sudden the room was full of people. They came from nowhere. Everyone from my office, where Misty had worked the last year also, had all come to visit her and the baby. What a good surprise! Everyone was smiling and happy, being very supportive. We had about eight or nine people in the room. They were all disappointed to hear that they could not hold Riley, but understood. We laughed and carried on for about an hour and they had to leave, but it was a good break.

Later that evening, Lisa came back up to the hospital room and catered in a bunch of food from Uncle Julio's. We had a lot of happy people by now. They loved the food and we got Misty and Brent to laugh for a while.

CHAPTER TWO

RILEY WAS KEPT IN NICU where they monitored everything: his respiration, his blood pressure and his bilirubin. He had marks on his little face from the tape to keep his oxygen tubing in place. They found he was allergic to the tape.

We had to be sterile before we could enter the NICU to see him. Our hands had to be scrubbed at the sink with special soap. We put on a mask and a robe before we entered the room. Then we went in to see him. Misty did this several times a day, as she was breast-feeding him. They discharged Misty three days after he was born.

After she was discharged, she had a very difficult time leaving her baby at the hospital and going home to rest. The nurses would tell her to go home and get the rest she needed and she just felt so guilty leaving him. Brent had to help her through this. It was difficult for both of them, and they just coaxed and encouraged each other as much as they could.

She told me she would just break down and sob uncontrollably once she got home. She just could not believe what was happening. Why?

It wasn't so much the fact that he might have Down syndrome at this point, as having to leave him at the hospital and come home to rest, and not knowing what or if something might happen.

It would get better, I assured her. The doctors and nurses would figure out what was going on with Riley and he would be home with her very soon. I had to keep reminding myself too. I kept thinking, *If I say it out loud, it might come true.*

We could hold him and rock him in the NICU, fighting all the tubing and wiring for the machines they had him hooked to. They had several rocking chairs in the unit.

Do you know that they have volunteers that come to just hold and rock the babies? I find that amazing. What a wonderful job.

Brent's dad and stepmother came in from Arkansas the weekend after Riley was born. His whole family lived in Arkansas, so it was hard for Brent without them for support. Everyone was glad to see Larry and Pat, and they were happy to meet their new grandson. They got to visit Riley in the NICU and hold him. They stayed for a couple days and also helped Misty and Brent as they were moving to Decatur, Texas. They agreed with me—he just did not look like a Down syndrome child. This was the first time I had met Brent's dad and step-mom. They seemed very nice and they got along great with Misty and Brent. Their visit was for the weekend, and the time passed way too quickly.

The doctors continued to be baffled by Riley's condition, not knowing what was causing his oxygen levels to fluctuate the way they did. They ran what seemed like a lot of tests and had all the monitors going, but it did not seem to tell them what they needed to know. That was the part I found difficult as the doctors really had no answers for our questions yet. It was hard to be patient. Why couldn't they figure out what was going on? I could not understand. They were educated for this purpose. I needed to know now.

Finally, after one week of being on oxygen and not getting stronger, it was determined that he should be transferred to the Cook's Children's Hospital where they were better equipped to diagnose his condition. This was kind of scary, as they were admitting they could not fix whatever it was and a bigger hospital might really find something serious. We were all very nervous. Riley was transferred by ambulance, accompanied by his mother.

I was at the hospital that afternoon as soon as I could get there. There he was in a little bassinet, hooked up again. The new place was much different than the other. It was overwhelming, the number of babies, the way it was arranged. The number of staff. You walked in to see rows of see-through bassinets with lots of equipment and wires hooked up to each one, and inside each was a little tiny human being lying there.

Within a few days of being at Cook's, the pulmonology doctor ordered a swallow study test. This had not been done yet. He thought something was going on with the way he swallowed fluids. Every time after he would nurse, his oxygen levels would fall dramatically and they figured out there might be a correlation. Within minutes of that test it was discovered that Riley was aspirating the liquids he was being fed into his lungs. Finally, after the tests were completed, the doctor advised it was his swallowing.

A simple treatment was all he had to prescribe. A thickener had to be added to any liquid given to Riley and that should alleviate the aspiration problem. They monitored him for a few more days and did other tests to make sure their diagnosis was correct. They were right, it was working, and Riley started getting better.

We were all still concerned about the holes in his heart and they said it could correct itself with time. It might not be as desperate as it sounded. They would just need to check on him frequently, but for us not to worry at that time. (Yeah right, not worry, that's a joke.)

Since Misty was breast-feeding, she would now have to milk herself, store it and mix it with a thickener. This was not optimal, as she would lose out on the close bonding that comes with breast-feeding. But her baby would be able to breathe on his own and that would make everything okay.

So, as luck would have it, our little Down syndrome boy basically had two little problems that could be corrected and that he might grow out of eventually. How lucky could we be? A large percentage of Down's children have other debilitating ailments, like vision problems, hearing problems, heart defects, gastrointestinal problems (digestive), and respiratory problems.

This facility was so amazing, especially the way they were set up to care for sick babies. What an eye opener. I had never known or been around anyone with a sick baby. I had been so fortunate. It was very clinical, stark, clean, white, technical, cluttered, and they had all the equipment and all the personnel. I was truly thankful and awed at their expertise.

Riley was still in Cook's over Halloween. The nurses got Misty and Brent to hold Riley in a plastic pumpkin for the cutest picture. There he was with his oxygen tube on his face, so little, propped up in a pumpkin with Mom and Dad. Then Cheyenne got to come in with his costume on and take a picture with his brother. Cheyenne told me how much he would love his little brother no matter what was wrong with him. He was a very loving little boy.

I was there every day to see my grandson, not knowing what would happen. I knew after that first day that our lives, our perceptions, our hopes and our dreams were all different. We had a special needs child in our family.

It did not stop there. Before Riley could be discharged, Misty and Brent had to go through a CPR class at the hospital. Also, they had to spend the night with him in a private room where they learned how to give him his breathing treatments with the nebulizer. The hospital staff wanted to make sure that the new parents were going home equipped to care for their special needs child. I got to be there with them for a lot of this; not all, but a lot.

The hospital did most of the referrals for assistance. They notified all the different agencies and let them know that Riley would need physical, occupational and speech therapy to begin with. Misty and Brent, as parents, would now need all the love and support that could be mustered. I knew that as the maternal grandmother, my role would be huge. I wanted to be their rock. I thought, *This wonderful couple, blessed with this beautiful boy, will have a hard time as it is, so I will do all I can to ease their burden as much as they will allow me.*

Well, eighteen days was long enough. On November 6, the doctors said okay.

Finally, Riley got to go home.

CHAPTER THREE

THE BABY'S ROOM WAS JUST adorable—primary colors and Mickey Mouse. But Mom and Dad had him sleep in their room. Even though they had the baby monitor and everything set up for him, they could not leave this little person by himself.

Misty found herself busy beyond words. From the first day home Riley was sleeping through the night, which was fabulous. He did not seem to cry a lot, although there were times he would cry out and no one could figure out why. The doctor gave them drops for his indigestion. They thought this might be causing some of the problem. It did seem to help. Everything had to be sterile as Riley would be more susceptible to any infections that might be around than a normal baby. Down syndrome babies have smaller airways, nasal passages, etc. So this too was cause for concern.

Riley loved taking his bath. He was very alert, looking around, kicking his feet. How, how could this be a Down syndrome baby? She would lay him on the floor and he would raise his head! He was looking around with his head up, on his belly, after being home for four days! That appeared to be normal development to me. I still had my doubts about his condition.

Riley was right there in the floor playing and every time I would come over, I would come at him with my fingers twitching and saying, "Here comes the tickle monster. The tickle monster is coming to get Riley," and he would start smiling and laughing and wiggling around. It was so cute. He was the most ticklish baby I had ever been around. He seemed to know me. I wanted him to know me, and I did not want to be a stranger to that little guy.

Misty was so good with him and she didn't even know it. She completely surrounded him with sounds, colors, textures…anything that might stimulate his mind or his gross motor skills. She spent time with him when he was awake, let him rest when he was asleep. They were finally developing a routine, a rhythm.

I was over there whenever I could get out for a while. I always had my camera. I even got her to the point that she kept her camera with film in it. With this kind of fragile beginning, it was important to me to record everything. What if things changed for the worse? It just was not the same as having a normal baby.

In November, I had to be gone for a week to see my grandmother in New York. I loved going to see my family there. They were supportive and compassionate and they too were dealing with a lot as my grandmother was in a nursing home with Alzheimer's. She was eighty-six years old and slowly going down hill. My time with her was more precious too.

Soon it was December, and it was time for his first cardiology appointment. We were all anxious to hear about the two holes in his heart. What kind of news would the doctor give us? We were all anxious.

Misty called me that afternoon all out of breath. "Mom, guess what? They're gone. Both holes closed up. His heart is just fine!"

I could not believe my ears. *How could we be so lucky? Are they kidding?* It was just too great. I was ecstatic.

If that wasn't enough, it was also time to go see the geneticist in December. Misty said she was a nice doctor. She did confirm that Riley had nondisjunction trisomy 21. That is where the cell division at the 21st chromosome resulted in three cells instead of two, and it is copied and transmitted to the other new cells, resulting in 47 chromosomes instead of 46. This is the most common type of Down syndrome. Ninety-five percent of all children with Down's have this type. This kind of Down syndrome is not inherited though. It occurs at the formation of the egg or the father's sperm. It is not passed along from one generation to the next. I did not know this. It really surprised me and everyone else.

Now it was time to accept his condition. It was what it was and nothing could be done to change it. He would have limited mental and physical capabilities. We would just have to make sure and prepare him as best we could for some type of life. I prayed I could do this as the grandmother. What if I just could not? I just was so unsure of everything, but I knew I had to be strong no matter what.

January came and I was glad that the year 2000 was gone. Riley was old enough now to begin physical therapy and occupational therapy at home. The therapists would come out to the house and work with Riley and Misty. She was instructed on how to continue the therapy after they left so that they might see progress. And they did start seeing progress. He seemed to learn very fast, he was so alert all the time.

I was there visiting one afternoon when one of the therapists showed up. She took out her toys and started talking with Riley. He just looked at her and smiled, cooing and playing. Then came a loud laugh. *What a sweet sound*, I thought.

That's when Misty remarked, "See there, my child has *Up syndrome*, not *Down syndrome!*"

We all just busted out laughing. How perfect, how true. This little guy that we were so scared of…and scared for…had brightened our lives already in the few months he had been alive. What a joy to be around. There I was constantly bringing out the camera, taking pictures again and again. Everyone would make fun of me being so click happy, but I couldn't help it. I wanted everyone to see what I saw.

Brent took great care with Riley Joe. He could get Riley to show us his sad face just by telling him, "Riley Joe, show me your sad face." Then he would say, "Good boy. Now show Daddy your happy face," and Riley would do it; he understood what his dad was telling him. They had developed a very special bond and Riley responded well to Brent.

Even though he was doing well, the visits to the different doctors were non-stop. They would have three to four doctors' visits one week and two to three therapy sessions the next week. He was growing at a slower rate than normal babies and this was considered normal. He still was not sitting up on his own and this was cumbersome in caring for him. The doctors would tell us not to worry, but of course we would anyway.

His hearing was tested and found to be better than average. This was why he became very upset when a loud sound would startle him. If there were a lot of people around visiting and laughing, if someone laughed loudly, or spoke in a loud voice or a deep voice, Riley would start crying.

A weekend invitation came to Misty and Brent in April, and I was going to get to keep Riley for a whole weekend. I was so excited. Misty and Brent needed to get away and finally they would let me have time with my grandson. I knew how to do his breathing treatments, I knew how to give him his stomach medicine, and I knew how to feed him. We were all set.

Riley and I and Bob had a blast. I had more fun than Bob as I was kind of selfish, keeping him to myself. I rocked him, held him, sang to him, read to him and played with him. When it came time to put him to bed, I went to bed with him. We had a playpen set up in the extra bedroom and there was a twin bed in there also. I did not let him out of my sight. He slept through the night. It was great. He was such a happy baby. He had one crying spell before he went to bed and after it was over, it was over. The weekend went by very fast and they came back on Sunday afternoon. The next week I was so sore from lifting him and bending to play—I was not used to it! I really did not care, I had fun.

CHAPTER FOUR

THE SECONDARY INSURANCE THAT THEY had for Riley was finally cancelled and the bills started piling up. It took a spreadsheet and my twenty years of health insurance claims examining to help them figure it all out. Unless you have someone that knows by experience how claims should be paid, you could end up paying bills you do not owe. I think it is outrageous that the insurance companies cannot be more helpful. It is sometimes the fault of the doctor's office not knowing what to do also, and their accounting department should be more educated on how claims are processed and paid, especially if there are two insurances.

Misty was also trying to do some telemarketing from home for my company. It worked okay for a little while, but she was not very successful. She was frustrated by that and the fact that it was difficult for her to estimate her time available when Riley did not need or want her attention. She and Brent needed the additional income, but it was just not working.

After a time, there was difficulty in keeping up with their regular bills on one income. Brent was working as much as he could, but it was not enough. They made too much to qualify for any government programs in Texas. They tried qualifying Riley for Supplemental Social Security. They had heard he might be eligible, but they kept running into road blocks. Government bureaucracy is not easy to deal with, as I am sure a lot of you know.

Misty maintained her routine with Riley through all of it. She was so frustrated with the rest of it, she just broke down one day with me. She was crying and putting herself down for not being able to work or bring money into their home. It was pitiful.

I told her, "You know, Misty, someday, when I grow up, I want to be just like you! You are my hero. You are handling all of this so well, taking care of this baby and you and Brent. Everything will fall into place eventually. You just have to have a little faith and some patience."

Misty was not good at faith or patience, she never had been. However, after awhile she calmed down and agreed with me, and then we hugged. I wanted so badly to take all of her pain away, if only I could.

Misty and Brent got through their financial problems together. They really did love each other and their son. Because of that love they were able to deal with whatever would come their way. They did continue to have problems financially, but it never affected the way they cared for Riley or each other. It was inspirational to be a part of their lives.

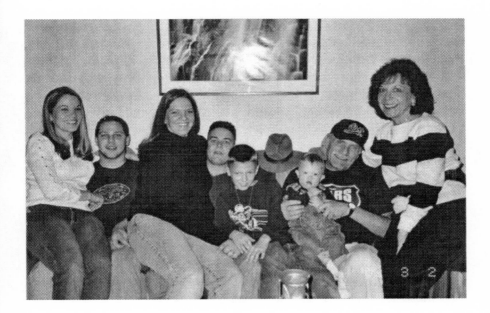

CHAPTER FIVE

MY GRANDMOTHER, CAROLINE BRIAMONTE, WHOM I was named for, died in April. She lived in upstate New York with my Aunt Jean, Uncle Paul Newman (not the actor, better looking) and cousin Lisa. She had been sick for a couple years with Alzheimer's. I had gone to visit at least two-three times a year for the past couple years as her health had really started to decline. I was trying to spend as much time with her as I could and fortunately I was able to afford the plane tickets and the time from work.

Misty, Heather, Riley and I went up for the funeral. We surprised everyone with Misty and Riley. They needed a good surprise. Everyone had been so depressed and Riley would liven things up a little. They were so happy to see them. It was a good surprise.

We stayed for a couple days to visit and everyone fell in love with Riley. It was a sad event we went to, but some good came of it. A lot of family got to see each other and it was good moral support for the loss. I laughed so much and so hard at lunch on the day of the funeral I thought my face was going to fall off. My Uncle George and my cousin Greg were deliriously funny. One line after the other. I thought my gut was going to bust open.

We got home and I tried to get back into the swing of things and just about the time I was feeling better about it all, my very good friend and business acquaintance, Caroline Lynch, died of cancer. She lived in a suburb of Salt Lake City. She had been such a good friend, and I had stayed with her on a couple of visits. What a nice family she had. She was going to be missed a lot.

I went to her funeral alone, but I was not alone when I got there. She died exactly one month after my grandmother and she was twenty years younger than my grandma. I was worried, since things happen in threes, that I would be the third Caroline, being twenty years younger than Caroline Lynch. But that was not to be the case.

Then came June that year with a vengeance. My mother was diagnosed with breast cancer for the second time in twelve years. She'd had a mastectomy the first time and was put on tamoxifin for five years and had not experienced any problems since. But there we were again and she was going to have to have another mastectomy and chemotherapy this time around.

My dad was devastated. He doted on my mother and could not stand for her to be sick or hurt or upset. Dad was strong for her though. He cared for her in every way. He cooked, cleaned, whatever she needed. Anyway, I was able to spend a lot of time with them during the illness, and I was strengthened and saddened at the same time. It was horrible watching her go through the chemo treatments and what they did to her. *My god, when will this year end!* I thought.

It was hard, because I loved my mother and desperately wanted to be with her, but at the same time, Riley was growing and doing new things every day and I wanted to be with him also. Needless to say it was stressful. I could not do everything and be everywhere, no matter what I wanted.

Then when we least expected it, Riley became mobile. He was about nine months old when he started crawling. He wasn't even sitting up on his own yet, but he could crawl. You should have seen it. He was crawling around like the wounded soldier. He dragged one leg behind him. Then he would stick his butt up in the air. We could not figure out if his right leg bothered him or if it was just not as dexterous or if it was just his way. The doctor checked him out and said he was fine. It was just his way of crawling.

Everywhere we went, if Riley was put down to crawl, he drew a crowd. It was the most unusual crawl anyone had ever seen. And once he was on the ground he would have so much fun, he could care less who was or wasn't around. He did not know me or his mother at those times. He was on his own little mission to crawl. People would stop and just bust out laughing. It was great fun to watch. That child was truly in his own world at times and it was mesmerizing.

We would go shopping and people would stop and stare at him. Then Misty would have him do his happy and sad face that Brent had taught him and we would all just laugh. It was like he was an entertainer. He loved showing his talent. When Misty had shopping to do, I would let Riley crawl

21

wherever he wanted and keep up with him while she got her shopping done. It was great exercise for me and him.

It was during that time that Misty also decided to start teaching Riley sign language. She knew she would have to learn, so she would learn a sign and then teach Riley. You know, it takes longer for Down syndrome children to verbalize, but it does not mean that they do not understand. Giving Riley another alternative to communicate was very perceptive of his mom. I learned as we went too, so that I could understand what Riley wanted or was trying to say.

He learned the signs quickly. Of course, he personalized them. They weren't exactly how they were supposed to be, but we knew what he meant. He learned "please," "thank you," "more," "drink," "music" and he was doing well.

I often wondered, *If he can understand these things they are teaching him, does it mean he will be more advanced mentally or will he still be challenged?* We just did not know yet, and this was so disconcerting. Being so close to the situation really does mess you up. You see things and start wondering if you see it because you love the person so much or if it really is something to be considered important. Either way, Riley was going to be taught, shown and loved as long as his family was breathing.

It was in July when the therapist noticed the shape of Riley's skull. She showed us where his head was flat on one side, probably from the way he slept and the fact that he still was not sitting up on his own. Misty took him for an evaluation and it was determined that he had positional plagiocephaly, which is occipital flattening. It was suggested that a doc helmet being worn twenty-two hours of the day for four or five months to correct the condition. The insurance would cover most of the $3,000, but Misty and Brent needed to come up with a little over $300. That was not something they had set aside.

Misty got the bright idea to ask other family members for a small donation, like a charity. She figured if everyone could pitch in $5-$20 each, then it wouldn't be a burden on any one person. She called everyone and raised all the money for the helmet. I thought this was very creative of her to come up with the idea. She knew she needed to get the helmet for her son and a little bit of money from everyone helped her achieve her goal. Riley got fitted for his helmet, got it and wore it as much as he and Mom could stand it. It was unsightly, but within weeks we were seeing a change.

Riley continued wearing the helmet and was making great progress. You could actually see the difference. His personality was unchanged by the uncomfortable thing on his head. Oh yes, he would tug at it, but he wore it like a champ.

CHAPTER SIX

MISTY HAD BEEN HAVING STOMACH pains for about six months and then in July, she went to the emergency room. Her stomach pain was so bad she could not handle it and had Brent take her to the hospital. This had happened a couple of other times over the past six months. They admitted her and the next day it was determined that her problem was with her gallbladder and they recommended immediate surgery.

I was appalled. How in the world could a twenty-four-year-old have a bad gallbladder or gallstones? They did emergency surgery on her the next afternoon and she did very well. They kept her in the hospital for five days and then finally sent her home.

Of course, she would not be able to lift Riley for a couple weeks. Brent stayed home for a few days to take care of her and Riley, and then I stayed with her for a few days. She recovered quickly but it was a very difficult time. The doctor told us that a lot of young women after having children were having gallbladder problems and it was becoming quite common. I thought this was an odd phenomenon.

Riley had a great summer as both of his brothers came to stay for a couple weeks. Misty's son Cheyenne and Brent's son Zachary both got to spend two weeks with the Hoofman family. It was a great experience for everyone. Of course Misty got to play referee during the day while Brent was at work, but she tried very hard to make certain they all had a good time. They went to the zoo, the water park and the amusement park. There was even time to visit with Momo and Bob for dinner and dessert a few times.

This was the first visit with Zachary, and he was a beautiful little boy with curly brown hair and a shy demeanor. He was four years old and Cheyenne was eight, tall, blonde and lanky. Cheyenne soon broke Zachary of his shyness, at least around family members. They got along great, and as little as Riley was, he wanted to be right there with them.

The summer was soon over and things started to slow down a little. Over the Labor Day holiday, Bob and I went to Darlington, South Carolina, to see the NASCAR race there. It was a thrill to be there. I had never been to a race, so I was excited. Darlington is out in the sticks, but it is pretty. It was nice to take a break from everything. I knew I needed to be away from everything and everyone for a short time.

We got home right before the 9-11-2001 tragedy. If our trip had been a week later, no telling what we would have gone through. We were lucky. Of course, just like everyone else, we were all freaked out. We talked about leaving the country, hiding out somewhere, just to get away from the fear.

With all that was going on, I finally decided I could not stand my bad habit another second. So, after thirty years of smoking cigarettes, I figured it was time to quit for good. I had tried several times before to give it up and just could not let go for good. This time I went to an acupuncturist and used the patch. My biggest fear with quitting was gaining weight, so the acupuncturist could help me with the cravings for cigarettes and the new taste of food. I knew my metabolism would slow down when I quit, so hopefully the combination of the patch and the acupuncture would work for good. I was scared, but determined.

Riley's birthday came around and he was finally able to sit up in his high chair with no assistance. I could not believe it—one year old. Misty and I invited everyone and everyone came. We packed the house. Riley just could not understand what was going on. He was totally confused. He seemed to like the presents and he really liked the cake and ice cream. It was limited to just birthday cake and gifts as anything else would have been too much for Misty and Brent to handle.

All the family members were there and it was great that everyone could get along as well as they did. It would make a difference in the attitudes of the children and their eventual outlook on life.

Misty started to introduce him to some solid foods a little at a time. She had to be careful he wouldn't choke. He seemed to like almost anything she gave him. Of course it was all baby food. She found he loved pudding as a snack. He loved ice cream and he would always sign for "more." So, as Momo, I tried to keep both on hand in case he was at my house and needed a snack.

You know most kids at that point are holding their spoon or fork or even their drink cup, but not Riley, not yet. He had to be fed his food and his drinks even at a year old. However, he could show you his sad face, happy face, the wave (with his hands), lizard (with his tongue) and understood direction. We had proof of that.

A few days after his birthday, I had gone shopping and found a Halloween costume that was just perfect for him. After I bought it, I was so excited I went over to see him right away. Misty and I put him in the costume and we both had our cameras out. The pictures came out perfect. In fact, I used one of them for my screensaver at work.

It was at that time that Brent decided to try a career change. He went from being a lineman for an electrical contractor to selling cars. He was ready to try something different and he put his whole being into it. He was determined that he would succeed. The first couple of months were rough for them, money wise, but then he got his groove and he soared like an eagle. He could definitely sell.

They were finally seeing some light at the end of their tunnel. Maybe things would go their way for a change. All they wanted was to be able to support themselves and have a little extra to set aside for a rainy day. There was a price however. He worked a lot of hours and that was not good for family life.

CHAPTER SEVEN

IT WAS TURNING COLD OUTSIDE and Misty and I found it was a great reason to shop. We found the cutest winter clothes for Riley. I had no idea some retailers had such great stuff. They have little tiny sweaters, caps, mittens and anything else, just cuter than I had ever seen before. How could a Momo resist? I really didn't want to resist.

It was November and he started pulling himself up on the coffee table. "Look at this!" Misty yelled.

I ran into the living room to see Riley smiling at me from the other side of the coffee table standing up on his little tiptoes. "Oh my God!" I cried. "When did he start doing this?"

"Just now!"

We just looked at each other and gasped. We could not believe it. Then we clapped for Riley. He loved for us to clap and then he would clap his hands.

This was going to get interesting. With him crawling and pulling up now, we would need to make sure things were out of his reach. He did not pay too much attention to the things that were within his reach, he just wanted to get around and get up. He was on his little mission again, only now it was focused on getting in an upright position.

He definitely had an advantage as he was wearing his helmet, so if he fell he had some protection. He was so full of energy. From the minute he got up it was nonstop with him, and he was not lethargic or lazy or slow. He was a boy on the move, and what was great to watch was he seemed to know.

Time was flying by as it usually does when you have children and it's the holidays. Some of the family came over to my house for Thanksgiving dinner. It was a nice day for visiting and eating. Misty and Brent with Riley, Heather and her boyfriend Troy, Misty's friend Jamie and her husband and baby, and my sister Marlene. Everyone that wanted got to hold Riley. My sister Marlene was just crazy over Riley, and she hugged and kissed and rocked him for a big part of the day. Of course it was a battle I did not give up easily. We were all stuffed by the day's end, but it was a beautiful day and being together with family and friends made it fabulous.

The long weekend made it nice for visiting. I was able to visit with Misty and Brent and Riley for a couple extra days. Bob was pretty flexible about us going over there so much. He and Brent got along great and they would have these ice cream eating contests, not per se, but they ate a lot of ice cream. It was hilarious because they would both really talk it up. Anyway, Misty and I just shook our heads. I would just look at ice cream and gain five pounds.

Misty's birthday came along in December and we got to babysit overnight. Riley was a little older and he now realized he was not with Mom and Dad. Even though he knew me well, he was not happy. After about two or three hours of crying, he settled in and started playing with me a little bit. I ended up letting him fall asleep in my arms before I put him to bed. It was good for Misty and Brent to have a break.

The winter came like a vengeance and the place that Misty and Brent were living was not built very well and they were starting to have problems keeping it warm. A few nights they all slept in front of the fireplace because it was too cold in the house for Riley. It was a problem that appeared was not going away easily. The fact that they were out in an area with no trees did not help.

Christmas day came and everyone gathered at my house for dinner. I always made a traditional holiday dinner. That year I wanted to have ham and turkey with all the fixings. We had food to last for hours for an army. We all squeezed in the dining room and had a great time.

Riley was starting to eat different foods and trying different drinks. It was fun watching his face as you would feed him different things. Misty also introduced him to the sippy cup. This was a cup with a spill-proof lid that he could sip from; however, he could not hold it on his own yet.

The presents were overflowing. The two grandsons were there along with Misty and Brent, Heather and Troy, my brother Craig, his wife Sharon and their two sons, Brian and Adam. It turned out to be a great day. Riley and Cheyenne were the best to watch opening their gifts and playing. Riley was not really sure about the present-opening process. He was somewhat standoffish about the whole ordeal, but we all made it okay for him. The weather was nice, so we were able to go outside for a while and enjoy the day even more. The day lasted forever and we all wallowed in it and got lazy as the afternoon wore on.

The next week we had the opportunity to have Riley overnight again. I was happy to keep him again. However, when the day came it did not appear he was too happy to have his parents leave him. We went through the sobbing again, which wasn't really crying, it was a pitiful sob. It lasted for a while and he finally fell asleep. I still could not get enough, I wanted to be around him all the time.

It was fun because Misty and Brent went to dinner with Heather and Troy. It was great that they all got along so well. It really warmed a mother's heart that her children were grown and still cared about the other. I knew that they would be there for each other no matter what happened.

CHAPTER EIGHT

THE PULMONOLOGIST HAD SCHEDULED A follow-up swallow study in January 2002 to see how Riley was progressing. Misty called all excited again. "Guess what?" she said. "Riley is all better. He isn't aspirating anymore. His swallow study showed everything is flowing the way it should. Can you believe it?"

"Wow," I said, "that is just too great. Is there anything else you have to do?"

She said, "No, just be careful and watch him for a while. Otherwise he can drink and eat like you and me."

What a great way to start the New Year, I thought. Things were going to be different this year, I just knew it. My plan to lick my smoking habit was working. I had not desired or had a cigarette in four months. Wohooooooooooooo!

The winter became unpredictable. One day in January, we had a very bad ice storm. It happens in our area of Texas a couple times a year. I left work early to try to miss the worst of it, and I did pretty good. However, Bob was not so lucky and neither was Brent. It took Bob three hours to get home safely, and Brent couldn't make it all the way home so he stopped off at our house and spent the night, which meant Misty and Riley would have to tough it alone.

The next morning was just as treacherous. Brent attempted to get home to Misty and Riley, and it took him another three hours to get home. Misty was out of her mind with worry. The bad weather really takes its toll down here in Texas. They do not have road equipment for that kind of weather, so all they can do is sand the streets. It is nerve racking if you commute any distance at all. But Brent wanted to be with his family, so he braved the bad roads.

They were still having problems with their home and the heating and it was getting ridiculous that they were sleeping in front of their fireplace. They started thinking they were going to have to move, possibly closer to town. They decided that they would start looking. If for no other reason than Riley was at risk in a home that could not be kept warm in the winter.

He woke up with a fever a few days later and the doctor determined that he had an ear infection and bronchitis. His airways were so small, it made him more susceptible to problems. Misty and Brent were up with him at night giving him breathing treatments to help alleviate his cough and ease his breathing. The antibiotic started to kick in and he was better, but they knew how the scenario would continue.

The cold months do not last very long in Texas and we were thankful for that fact now that Riley was around. It was difficult to get out and about with a little one in the cold weather. That would be true even if he was normal. He had always been good on car rides, that was never a problem, it was just getting to that point. We all managed to get through it and do whatever needed to be done, one thing at a time.

CHAPTER NINE

THEY FOUND A HOUSE IN Saginaw after looking for about two months. It was pretty nice, only a year old. Misty had grown up in Saginaw, so she would be comfortable there and it put Brent closer to his job. They moved in March and I watched Riley while they moved. Brent had been working so much that Misty did all of the packing and a lot of the moving without him. There's always a price for success and Brent was very successful at selling, but the hours were not family friendly.

The house was only fourteen miles from me. I clocked it and it took about twenty minutes to get there. I thought it was great. I was very excited for them moving closer to me. The house gave Riley plenty of running-around room. It did not take him long to check it out. Misty baby-proofed the house, so Riley could go anywhere his little body would take him.

I would stop by to visit them right after getting home from work, and she would be doing something in one room and Riley would be off by himself somewhere playing. Of course she always knew where, but it was great that there were no obstacles for him to endure. Usually he was in his room listening to music or pulling his toys out everywhere. Typical behavior for a baby his age, I thought. But he loved his music. He would dance around and try to clap his hands, he would just get very excited.

He still took a nap every day and this gave Misty some time to breathe. She could do what she wanted without worry, if only for an hour. She was beginning to get restless being at home with Riley for so long. She was used to being around people. Misty was definitely a people person. If you spent more than five minutes with Misty you knew her life history and her goals and you knew she was not a story teller. She told you how it was and she usually did not hold back.

Brent was definitely starting to see the results of his hard work. His sales ability was showing up in his paychecks, and he made salesman of the month four months in a row. I was ecstatic for them, thinking this would be their life, yea right! Not.

It was around April when Cheyenne had his ninth birthday; my goodness where had all those years gone? Misty started hearing rumblings that Jeremy and Karen were not getting along. There was the incident where Jeremy was hurt on the job and then he was terminated, then he was laid off. Finally in May we heard that they were splitting up. Well, this meant Cheyenne would be uprooted from his current home to move out with his dad to an apartment. Then Misty found out he was being left alone. That did not make her happy and she let Jeremy know. He then started to leave Cheyenne with Misty.

It was soon suspected that maybe Jeremy was doing drugs and alcohol again. Misty was so concerned she contacted a lawyer to find out if she had any options. Well, there was definitely a possibility according to the lawyer. Hope started springing up all over the place. It would be a dream come true for Misty to have her son with her again. Yes, he had been happy with his dad over the last five years, but it was hard for Misty not to have a say in some of his upbringing.

After going to court three times, Jeremy being subjected to a hair follicle drug test, and him not showing up for two subsequent court dates, full custody of Cheyenne was turned over to Misty. Of course this was a double-edged sword as we would soon discover. As happy as we were about it and thought Cheyenne was happy, this was not the case. It would be a rather long and difficult adjustment for both Cheyenne and Misty. But as the old saying goes, anything worth having does not come easily.

The boys got along for the most part and Misty could not be happier about that fact. However, she still wanted to get out and be more productive, so she landed a job as a medical assistant at a local hospital. The hours were flexible and she found a brand-new daycare associated with the hospital right nearby that would take Riley Joe. Cheyenne only had a few weeks before school started, so he stayed some with Karen and some with Karen's mother; they both loved him beyond words and we all knew he missed his life.

It was July and Riley was now twenty-one months old. He finally started pulling up to the coffee tables to steady himself and then just stand there. He did this for a couple weeks and then one day he just stood there not holding onto anything. A week later he took his first step and he has yet to slow down. For about a month he did his walk crawl combo, which was pretty hilarious. He looked like he would tip over because his feet are different. I don't know how to describe them. They are flat, but he walks on the outside of them and the big toe has a big space between the next toe. It just looks as though he should not be able to walk on them. So when he did, he deserved a celebration.

The second time he went to daycare he got sick with an ear infection. He started running a fever while at the daycare, so Misty called me to pick him up. Then she had to take him to the doctor as soon as she got off work. I thought this was not a good sign of things to come, but Misty really wanted to make a go of it, maybe it was just a routine thing that happens to all kids when they are exposed to other kids.

Riley was started on the antibiotics and he started feeling better, so the next week Misty dropped him off at the daycare. He did alright for the next three days that Misty worked. The week after, she called me at work and asked me to pick him up on my way home as he was not feeling well and he was running a fever. I loved picking him up.

If he wasn't feeling too bad, we had great fun when it was just the two of us. We would race through the house, turn on his CD player, dance and play with all his toys. This went on for a few weeks with him being sick, getting well, going back to daycare and getting sick again. It was almost too much for all of us, but then one Sunday morning, Misty called from work. She had hurt her back putting a patient in his bed from his wheelchair. She could barely move.

I raced over there to see what I could do to help, but Brent had it all under control. Misty was in bed on muscle relaxers and the boys were playing, so I cooked them all breakfast. This woke Misty up. She loved my breakfasts and she ate and went back to bed. We did not know it yet, but that was the end of her working career for a while. It was for the best, as Riley could not handle daycare at that point, maybe later.

CHAPTER TEN

SUMMER WAS OVER FOR CHEYENNE and it was not much of a summer for him. He had lost his home, his dad, his whole world. He started school in Saginaw and it was not fun for him or Misty. They both struggled, and Brent with them, because Cheyenne had not had much discipline in his life and Misty and Brent knew it was needed. Times were changing for Cheyenne and it would be a struggle.

Riley and Cheyenne got along like most brothers. They had good days and bad days. They could play for hours on the good days, with Cheyenne teaching and challenging Riley. They chased each other and they roughhoused with each other. It looked like it was going to be a good fit. Even though Cheyenne could be self-centered, you could see him struggling through that when it came to Riley. For instance, wanting desperately to play with Cheyenne's PlayStation, Riley came in his room, stood in front of him, grabbed for the control and Cheyenne was patient until Riley got bored. Other times it was quite the opposite. But for a nine-year-old he handled his brother with love and compassion.

Then came Riley's second birthday. Misty planned a nice party. There were about forty people that came—relatives, neighbors and co-workers. It would just be a snack and cake party as Riley was still unsure of the gift opening and the crowd of people. He did finally relax a little after the presents were opened and he got time to play.

The cake at the end of the party was hilarious. Riley really dug into it that year and had blue icing all over the place. He was walking pretty good at that point and he was not afraid to do anything or go anywhere where there were other kids. He seemed very open to socializing with others, which I thought was a good sign. He seemed to demonstrate all the normal qualities of a two-year-old. How could he be anything but normal?

That year at Thanksgiving, we had my mom and dad, as well as Heather and Troy, Misty, Brent, Cheyenne and Riley and my business partner Lisa, who brought her significant other, Annette. I tried cooking my turkey in a new electric roaster that year and it was a disaster. I had never messed up a turkey before. Do not follow the directions on those roasters, they are wrong. Anyway, it turned out fine as I had a fried turkey also. So, while we cooked the other turkey longer (in the regular oven), we devoured the fried one.

It was a good day. The weather was perfect and everyone had a great time visiting. Mom was there with her cute straw hat on as she had lost all of her hair by that time. She and Dad seemed to have a good time. They all had plenty to eat and then there was dessert. We had lots of desserts and coffee. By the end of the day there was barely anything left to wrap up.

Riley was happy as soon as we put food in front of him. He loved to eat, but just like any other kid there were some things he did not like. He was not yet a meat eater, although he loved hot dogs, and he really liked potatoes and salad of all things. The dessert was his favorite thing. No way could you eat ice cream without sharing, or pudding for that matter. He would eat that stuff until he was sick, literally.

He was all over the house that day. He explored all the rooms (like he had never been there before) and went to just about everyone there that day. He especially loved the toy box I kept for him. We pulled that out and had toys all over the place. Bob even sat down with him to play with one of his toys. It was one of those days that just kept on going like it would last forever.

Of course the football game was on. We had to watch the Dallas Cowboys play and they always played on Thanksgiving Day. Sports always prompted the noise level to move up a notch or two, and it wasn't just the guys either. Riley was actually to a point where the noise did not bother him as much. He was back and forth in front of everyone vying for attention. Troy put his hat on him and he played with that for at least fifteen minutes. He had the room in an uproar with his antics and the hat. I know he knew what he was doing, he had to. It was a good sound no matter what. Riley was starting to develop a personality and it was fun to watch how he acted and reacted during gatherings.

That weekend we went shopping as Misty had a neighbor that was not going to have a very good Christmas for their three boys as money was not there. So she and I went to the toy store and played Santa. It was a lot of fun and Riley was having fun just running around the store when we let him. The toys got delivered to the neighbor and the boys never knew where they came from. It was fun just being together with Misty and the boys.

Christmas was fast upon us and I had all of my shopping done early, so the boys were not deprived of much. I tried not to go overboard, but really what is overboard?

That Christmas would be special, not only because we had Riley, but also, Mom was still with us and it was hard not knowing what could be in our future where she was concerned. There was a crowd that year. We had seventeen all together. I set up two tables to fit everyone. Oh, there was plenty of food—ham, turkey, dressing, potatoes, gravy, corn, green bean casserole, fried cauliflower, salad, cranberry sauce, rolls and drinks and, no, we did not forget the desserts. Cheyenne and Riley had fun opening presents from everyone. Riley was a little less cautious but still not as excited as he would be in a couple more years. And that year, Misty and Brent bought us a video camera and I put it to use immediately. I captured the whole group all day long…what fun.

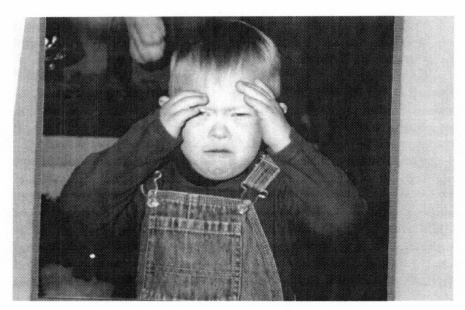

CHAPTER ELEVEN

THE NEW YEAR (2003) STARTED off with Misty telling me that they were going to look into the probability of moving to Arkansas. Brent was from there and his five-year-old son lived there with his ex-wife. He and Misty were concerned that he was not getting the influence of a stable father figure that he so desperately needed. His shy demeanor had become almost debilitating, and Brent felt responsible because he had not had an active role in his son's life up to that point.

I heard what they were saying, I just could not comprehend the possibility of my best friend and my grandsons leaving me to move off somewhere. How in the world could I live through that ordeal? Now I was very worried about me.

It is amazing how your mind can let you block something out for a while, and you just go on about your business without thinking about that something. That is just how I made it through. What in the world was I thinking though? No matter what, or how I tried to deal with it, I would still have to face it eventually.

Riley was becoming more independent and dependent if that makes sense. In his familiar environment, he was very independent, surrounded by music, color and different shapes, forms and textures. Misty always made sure it was accessible to him and organized for him. He still was not talking, but he understood everything going on around him. He would let you know if he was hungry or thirsty by signing. He rarely whined about it or cried. He was the happiest little guy when he was eating, he loved to eat. However, we all tried to be cognizant of what happens with a lot of Down's children. They do not understand being full and that is why they are, more often than not, overweight.

What Misty tried to do was keep healthy and fun snacks for Riley to eat. If the fun snacks came in low fat, that is what she would buy. She tried to round out his diet, but that was difficult when he would not eat just anything. The therapists that were visiting Riley on a regular basis helped her with nutritional information and guidance. His therapists were gems, the nicest, most compassionate human beings I ever met. However, Texas did not seem to offer much more than the therapists coming to visit. I know of one school in the area that cost about $8,000 per school year. They offered scholarships and Misty filled out the paperwork even though it looked as though they were moving, just in case.

Riley and Cheyenne were doing well together at that point. Riley wanted to be with him all the time. I think that was the reason that Misty obtained custody of Cheyenne. He was meant to be there for Riley. He did a lot for Riley, playing with him, reading to him, horsing around with him. In fact, if the boys were with me, and Misty was away, I could always count on Cheyenne to help me out when it came to Riley. The neighborhood kids would come over and want to play with Riley also. The girls loved it when he was outside playing, because he was someone they could mother. Riley would go along with that for a while, but he had his own agenda. He was, in fact, a person with a mind and opinion and his own way. That was the hardest thing for a lot of us to realize and remember.

The end of January, Misty and Brent wanted to visit Arkansas to see if there was work available for Brent, and also what the housing situation was like. They asked me to come stay at the house and keep Riley and Cheyenne so that they could go and do what needed to be done and come right home without the distraction of the boys. I was more than happy to spend a weekend with the boys.

What a blast we had. From having breakfast together to playing in the tub, to going out for a walk. We played, read, played and ate. I took pictures and shared them with everyone. Riley did really well with me. I was so afraid he would feel abandoned and mope all weekend, but he did not. We stayed busy and he loved it. He had so much energy. Cheyenne was there as a support to me and we also had alone time when Riley napped. But Cheyenne really liked going to play with his friends, so he was gone some of the time.

The weekend soon came to an end and I was sad to see it go. Misty and Brent came home refreshed and tired at the same time. They were excited about the prospect of moving and possibly starting fresh. They knew it would be different, but the unknown did not scare them much. They knew his family would be there to support them, so they kept up their positive attitudes and moved forward. Their trip had proven fruitful as it appeared they had found a place to live and Brent had three job prospects.

Misty was excited also because Arkansas offered more in the way of education for Riley. It was possible he could get into a school at his young age. They would have to live there before she would know for sure what they would qualify for, but it was more than he had available in Texas.

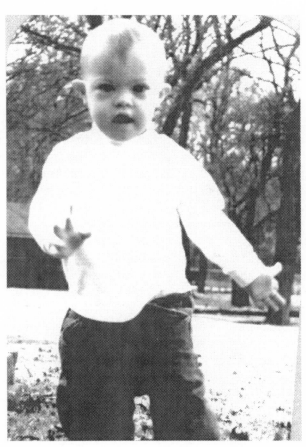

CHAPTER TWELVE

AS MISTY AND BRENT WERE dealing with moving and making a big change, it appeared Heather and Troy were also headed down a new road. Heather and Troy became engaged the first week of February. They had gone to San Antonio for a weekend getaway the first week of February in celebration of Troy's birthday. He had told us he was going to pop the question and had recruited help with the ring from me and his mom. He was going to wait until Valentine's Day but decided it would be more of a surprise if he did it that weekend. So they were at a park and he turned to Heather and asked her the question. She was so surprised and ecstatic, she told us later. We were all very happy for the two of them. They seemed to be good for each other and got along well most of the time. They were not ready to set a date as Heather still had to finish her education, but we decided quickly to have an engagement party. It would be something fun to distract us from the reality of Misty, Brent, Cheyenne and Riley moving to Arkansas.

We thought it would be a distraction...well, it was, but we still were stuck facing the fact that Misty would not be there the whole time to help us. So we decided to go ahead and plan a going-away party in March for the Hoofmans first and then we would have the engagement party for Heather and Troy in April. We wouldn't be too busy, would we?

Misty got started on her huge task by getting herself organized, and then by sorting out what she would take and what she would not. Then she decided she would have a huge garage sale. Riley seemed oblivious to what was going on, but he was two and a half, he was not supposed to know what was going on.

I was over there almost every day, seeing what I could do to help and visiting Riley and Cheyenne. Riley and I had such a good routine going together, it was wonderful. We played together, read books, danced and ate together. It finally was feeling like he really knew who I was, that I was an important person in his life and I would always be there for him. It felt great and I was so scared that now it was going to go away and we would never have that again.

His size really came into focus when a neighbor came over with her son who was almost a year younger than Riley and he was bigger. He was talking and he could do more physically. It was hard to see that kind of obvious comparison. What was even tougher was not talking about it when it was right there in front of you. Who wanted to upset Misty, or me for that matter, by talking about something that could not be changed? It was scary to talk about the obvious. Nobody wanted to come across negative. So we handled it the best way we could and sometimes that meant not saying anything at all.

The going-away party was huge. We had lots of people come by to say goodbye and wish good luck to Misty and Brent. There were several that showed up whom we had not seen in many years. It was funny because for such a sad event, we all had a great time.

Riley put on a show for us with a balloon. It was hilarious. He was chasing around a balloon that was stuck to his overalls. I caught it live on video, I am so glad I did. He would chase the balloon, fall down with the balloon, hit the balloon, and laugh at the balloon. He had everyone in the room laughing hysterically.

Anyway, after lots of food and lots of drink, the day wore on and all the goodbyes were said. The next weekend they would be heading out to Arkansas for good and my heart ached and to this day it hurts.

The garage sale went so well for Misty. She sold just about everything she wanted to and for about as much as she was asking for at the same time. I never had that kind of luck when it came to garage sales, that's why I would never have one, too much work for too little pay. The weekend went fast and it was all quickly cleaned up and put away or thrown away.

She and Brent packed up the U-Haul pretty much by themselves. It was all a tight fit, even after having the garage sale. Packing up your life and moving away on so many if's and questions lingering took a lot of guts, and Misty and Brent had a lot of guts. After they were through cleaning up the house, they came and spent their final night in town with me and Bob. The next day, we all got up and I was going with them to help them move and unpack and watch Riley for them.

It was as dreary a ride as I expected it would be, but it went by so very quickly. The boys slept most of the way. Cheyenne rode with Brent in the U-Haul, and Riley rode with me and Misty in the Durango. By time we stopped for breakfast, we were over halfway there. It was simply a matter of tolerance in that case. How much dread and dull could we tolerate before going crazy driving to that new place? We were there in no time. It was only a six-hour drive.

Most of Brent's family was at the house when we arrived, ready to help them unload and unpack. His dad, two of his sisters, his brother and their spouses and then the three of us and the two boys. We got that truck unloaded in record time. It was phenomenal. When it was done, the exhaustion set in immediately. What a day! I never slept so well.

The next two days I helped unpack, put together, wash, sort and clean. It was tiring and exhilarating at the same time. Riley would keep me distracted for a while and I would try to keep him busy. He loved dancing to his music in his room, so we would hide out in there to get away from it all. Amazingly we did get away from it all and it really felt like Riley and I were bonded for life and it was all I wanted. Surely he would remember me if I did not see him for a month or two...that was the scary part to me. I knew Misty, Brent and Cheyenne would be okay. It was Riley remembering his momo!

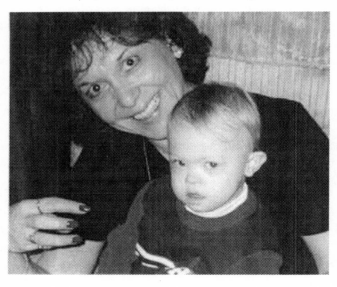

CHAPTER THIRTEEN

GOING HOME ON THE PLANE was very scary for me. I was leaving all my reasons for living every day. Oh, I know I had a husband, another terrific daughter, a business, etc. It just would not be the same or give me the satisfaction or enjoyment or fulfillment that had been there for me with Riley Joe. What if he didn't remember me when I came back? What if he got sick and I wasn't there? What if Misty realized she did not need me and told me she did not want me to visit so often? What if I got on Brent's nerves and he was glad I did not live nearby? Oh my.

Life was different now and I soon realized that I had to figure out a way to cope and stay busy. I would also have to visit so very often.

April rolled around and it was time for the engagement party. I had decided to have someone else cater it as it was just too many people for me to cook or prepare for. Heather and Troy had many friends and family they wanted to invite and I wanted them to have whomever they wanted and have plenty to eat and drink. So, I ended up with a great place, Central Market. They did a fabulous job and it was pretty reasonable.

The party was on a Sunday, and Misty and the boys came in for the weekend. We planned to go to Scarborough Fair on Saturday with all the people I work with that Misty knew, and we took Riley with us. He had a blast. There was a petting zoo there and he was awestruck with all the animals. He loved looking at and touching some of those animals, not all of them. It was a riot to watch him.

We all lasted about three hours and that was all the heat any of us could take, so we drove back to the house. When we got there, we decided we needed manicures and pedicures, so we got a hold of Heather and we all met at the Grapevine Mills Mall for some pampering. We took Riley with us and brought the stroller. The nail shop was pretty empty so we all sat at the pedicure spas together and Riley next to me in the stroller. We were cutting up having a good time and I looked over at Riley and he was putting his foot in his mouth.

I said to Misty and Heather, "Look, Riley is having himself a pedicure along with us." Well they both just busted out laughing and so did the staff there and I chimed in. Riley looked at us, and as if he knew we were laughing at him, he just started crying. I felt so bad. I hated that I had made him cry. I just did not realize how he must have felt scared.

Well, the engagement party was a huge success. There must have been at least one hundred people show up at the party. Heather and Troy had a great time and so did Bob and I. Troy's parents were there and they seemed to be very nice people. It was hard to have too long of a conversation with them as everyone was vying for their attention.

Misty enjoyed herself tremendously and Riley had a fairly good time. Part of the time he was tired and part of the time it was a little too noisy for his little ears. Loud areas or noises really bothered Riley.

Heather and I decided we would drive to Arkansas for Mother's Day in May. We left on Friday afternoon and arrived around eight that night. It was so good to see Misty and the boys again. Riley was a hoot and had learned some new signs. Misty and Heather wanted to learn how to make my manicotti, so Saturday morning we got up and started cooking.

We brought out the video camera and Misty turned on the radio. Riley was dancing while we were cooking. It was a great time. Life was appreciated by all of us at that time. We knew we had to savor every moment we had together.

After starting the dinner, we left to do a little shopping. It was always fun for us girls to go shopping. They would vie for my credit card to get something new. It was so much fun. Riley really loved shopping. He would grab hold of anything on the racks he could reach or he would be out of the stroller running wherever we would let him free. Cheyenne always wanted something new. He loved the mall. We all had a wonderful visit that Mother's Day weekend and it ended all too quickly.

Shortly after living in Arkansas, Riley was accepted at the Sunshine School, a program that provides for educational, physical and occupational therapy through state-subsidized agencies. He would start school in August at two years old and be in a class of five special needs children for six hours a day, five days a week. It would be very good for him to help him get a head start. Meanwhile, he would receive physical and occupational therapy at home until school started. He would be the youngest student on campus.

He was tested prior to school beginning in August, and receiving the results of those tests was not easy. It would be the first time we had any idea of his status. Misty was not prepared and neither was I as the news was poignant. Our Riley Joe, almost three years old, was basically at the level of an eighteen-month-old. That was it. That was the way it would be and we would have to get our arms around it and accept it and deal with it....that was the hard part.

I am sure it will get easier, then it will get harder, then it will get easier. Riley will grow and get smarter. He will progress and he will talk. I will get to watch his progression and be a part of it in all aspects. Of course, life has no guarantees, so this was speculative hope.

CHAPTER FOURTEEN

IT WAS AUGUST, TIME FOR school to start. Cheyenne was ready and now it was time to get Riley ready....ooh, that would be something. Misty got him a little backpack and I bought him his first-day-of-school outfit. It was momentous. At the Sunshine School, he would be in a classroom with four other students. Two of them also had Down syndrome. Rachel would be there. He knew her. She was four and blonde and cute as a button. Her mom and Misty and I, with Rachel and Riley, were the first ones there that first morning. I was armed with my video camera and my 35mm camera....had to have both.

Finally, the teacher and her assistant arrived and we were allowed to stay as long as we wanted. Riley went to every play station. He was totally taken in with all the toys, activities, etc. You could see he was excited. The other children arrived, two in wheelchairs. Yes, this was where he would be for a while, and we knew he was lucky to be here with such talented instructors. We snuck out after about two hours and he did not even notice. Later on that day when we went back to pick him up, he was so happy to see us. He ran over to Misty and hugged her neck, and then he came over to me and gave me a kiss. It was the end of his first day and everyone did well.

Cheyenne was adjusting to a new school also and his first day went pretty well for a fifth grade student. He thought he would like it just fine and he said everyone was pretty nice to him. I got video and pictures of him also, but he was a lot less camera ready than Mr. Riley.

I don't know why, but I just did not feel like Cheyenne was in a good place yet. I think he still had some hurdles to overcome.

Misty and Brent were embarking on another chapter of their life together and they did not even know it yet. They had found a new church home at Valley Baptist, and Bob and I went with them to church while we were there and Cheyenne decided it was time he was baptized. After all, he was ten years old and he knew right from wrong.

So after services we watched as Cheyenne was baptized and accepted responsibility for himself from that point forward. I thought he was too young, but it was not my call. Riley watched and clapped as his brother went forward. He loved his "bubby" so much, you could see how they interacted as brothers. It was beautiful. It was such a fabulous day. We celebrated afterwards and went out to dinner as it seemed like the right thing to do.

Time flew as usual and it was time for Bob and I to go home and I was sad again to leave. Misty and I cried, but knew we would see each other in about a month.

Riley did well at Sunshine School. They all loved him there, and he was considered very physically active for a Down syndrome child, as they are usually more lethargic due to low muscle tone. The therapists battled for his attention. They all wanted to work with Riley, since he was a very happy and active child. That kind of news was good to hear. We did not know how far it would take him, we would just have to wait and see, but each day seemed to be a little brighter than the day before.

It was September and I was having surgery, which made everyone nervous, but it was an uneventful hysterectomy and no complications. I recovered quickly and was glad to have it done. Heather helped me out at home quite a bit, bringing over food and making sure Bob and I had everything we needed. It is so amazing when your children come through for you and you think you might have done okay raising them. Troy's parents, along with Heather and Troy, showed up that next Saturday afternoon with food for everyone. I was half in and half out, still being on pain medicine, but I do remember thinking how thoughtful that was for them to think of us.

Of course, Misty and the boys came down the following weekend and spent time with me just to make sure I was alright. That was so great. It does make a difference in recovery time, believe me. She pitched in and cleaned the house for us. She was a whiz-kid when it came to cleaning. Both the girls being there for me and visiting with the grandchildren helped me more than anyone will ever know. But the time flew as I was not my normal self and I could not run after Riley or pick him up, that was tough not to do.

CHAPTER FIFTEEN

SOON IT WAS OCTOBER AND Riley was about to turn three years old. Where had the time gone?

I flew to Arkansas for the birthday party preparation. It was so great. I got off the plane and walked down the ramp to get past security where I knew Misty and the boys were waiting for me and then they saw me. All of a sudden, Riley ran up to me and jumped in my arms.

Oh my....

I swear I wanted to break down and get hysterical, but no, I had to keep it together so I would not scare him. Can you believe he actually remembered me? I could not believe it, I must have been dreaming.

Well, we were going to have his party at a community center where Misty had reserved a room. For snack foods, she wanted me to make my hot sauce and sandwich loaves, which are really simple with frozen bread dough. You just thaw and let it rise and then make fresh-type sandwiches. She also had a huge cake and ice cream and drinks.

The party was on Saturday and by two the place was packed with family and friends. Heather and Troy drove in and so did one of Misty's good friends, Jaime, from Fort Worth. Brent's sister Lori and her family and his brother and his family were also there, but I was the only grandparent.

Riley really had a lot of friends and family that were there for his party and, of course, I had my camera and video to record it all. Riley really had a good time with everyone there. His cousins and friends that came...he was hammin' it up. He really liked listening to music and dancing and he had started playing with little toy action figures. He would talk to them and play act with them and they liked the music as well. He had enough new toys and clothes to stock any young boy's room. He was lucky and we all knew it.

Misty was so excited. She was sure now that he would have enough clothes to last him through the winter. The toys were a real plus. Even though he had not outgrown all of his toys, he tired of them. That was one the realities we all needed to accept. At his party he received so many wonderful gifts. We truly had a fun time with Riley opening the gifts and then oohhing and ahhhhing over them. He giggled over that.

One of the difficulties you face with a special child is that sometimes the age level indicated on the package does not necessarily apply to your child. You have to know what your child is capable of and what he is not capable of. It is hard for those that really do not know, and those that do, but…! It was still fun and everyone seemed to enjoy the time we all had together along with the food.

The day ended and Sunday was upon us. I went to church with Misty and Brent and it was terrific. Riley went to the nursery where "grandma" watched over the little ones. She loved the babies and she loved Riley, you could tell. He went right on in. He obviously thought it was an okay place to be or he would have let everyone know he did not. Everyone at Valley Baptist, by that time, knew Riley Joe. He had been the hit of the party a few times they had fellowship dinners or devotionals with his shy demeanor. I was happy that they all loved him here, but at the same time I could not help but feel a little jealous that they got to spend time with Riley when I could not. It seemed unfair. I know I was being silly, but I just could not help it.

Well, after church we went to lunch and then on a drive to some scenic areas around Searcy. I had no idea it was so beautiful there. We drove over to a lake with a dam on one side. There were people fishing in the shallow end and it looked as though they were fly fishing. It was a beautiful scene in October with the leaves changing colors. We all took turns to get out and look around as Riley and Cheyenne had fallen asleep in the car.

Time flew and we were at the airport in no time. I just had them drop me at the front so I would not have to say goodbye or start crying.

I knew we would get together soon, we had to, it was almost like an addiction. I had to have my "Riley fix" and Misty had to have her "Mommy fix." My flight back was uneventful, thank goodness, and I was home in less than an hour.

It was hard sometimes to stay concentrated at work. With the economic times of my business and the agony over not being with all the people I loved, my days were long. But I kept going because I knew there was a little somebody that was as innocent as could be and would always be that way and I wanted to be around him. Misty and Brent were still struggling financially. They would get ahead for a while and something would happen to put them behind the eight ball. It seemed to be a constant battle.

Thanksgiving came and for the first time in many years I would not be cooking. Bob and I would go with Heather and Troy to his parents' home for the day. I made a fresh fruit basket cut out of a watermelon and then filled it with different fruits. It turned out great and was a lot of fun to make. We had a very nice day visiting and eating, watching movies and eating again and then there was dessert! Mmmmm. That is all I have to say about that.

Heather and I decided it would be great fun to surprise Misty with a visit on her birthday, which is December 11, so we decided to go the weekend before her birthday as her birthday was on a work day. We conspired with Brent to keep her home and busy. We left Dallas about five in the evening and arrived in Searcy around eleven. Brent was up to let us in and we bounced in to wake her up in bed and she was so happy to see us. It was fun to see her face.

The next morning we were awakened by a little squeal and a nudge. Riley Joe was there on the bed. What a cutie pie to wake up to. He was snuggling and then he got down from the bed and just looked up at me and I knew what he wanted. I positioned my hand in front of him all curled up and ready to dart into action and I was up in a minute and Riley shot out like a cannon and I was right behind him yelling, "Here comes the tickle monster....Here I come," and he was just a giggling the whole time. After ten minutes of that running around, Momo was done. We all finally took our showers and got ready for a big day of shopping.

We went out to breakfast for her first birthday treat and then we drove on down to Little Rock to shop their mall. We shopped and laughed and shopped some more. Riley loved going in and out of the stores as he knew Momo would rescue him from the stroller and let him walk and run for a while. We got home with all our packages and all in one piece. It was amazing. We were exhausted from all the shopping, it was hard work. Riley had fallen asleep on the way home and he was still asleep, but we knew he was going to wake up in a little while.

CHAPTER SIXTEEN

THE HOLIDAY PRESSURE WAS IN full gear and everyone was feeling the pinch. Misty and Brent were still living on a hope and a prayer and coming up short. Life was pretty difficult when it came to meeting those expenses, and coming up with money for extras was a little too much to comprehend.

Riley was doing well at Sunshine School and the local Kiwanis put on a Christmas lunch every year for the school. That year was no different and there was food, presents and Santa. Well, it was a great time for Riley. He loved it all, and even the Santa was fun for Riley. The local paper was there and Riley Joe's smile was on the second page of the paper and it was about half the page. Misty called me all excited. She just could not believe they put his picture, so big in the paper. But with his smile it was no wonder. The school had two or three Christmas events and Riley had a great time with everyone.

Brent and Misty were getting ready to come to Texas for Christmas, and they were frantically putting it all together as they would also have Zachary with them. Then Misty called me a couple days before they were supposed to leave, and she'd had to rush Cheyenne to the emergency room as he had broken both wrists when he had fallen off some swings. Mr. Show-off was trying to do something he probably should not have and had fallen backwards out of the swing and tried to cushion his fall by putting both hands down. Consequently, he ended up in two casts, one on each arm. It was pitiful!

They arrived late on Christmas Eve. It was wonderful to see them through my tired eyes. We got everyone situated quickly so that we could all get some sleep.

The next morning was terrific. Riley rose early and was up and around, hugging everyone and giving kisses for free. Heather and Troy came over early, as did Megan. We got breakfast out of the way quickly so that we could get to the presents. After all, the reason for Christmas was there. The house was quickly way too small with all the paper and gifts everywhere. It made it challenging to maneuver through the kitchen and cook dinner at the same time. Marlene and TW, her son, came as well as Craig, Sharon, Brian and Adam. It was so worth the effort. It was a very satisfying and enjoyable time. The fun and the laughter and the love inside that house was overwhelming to me, I could barely contain myself.

Later on in the evening Cheyenne's grandpa from his daddy's side of the family came. He was so happy to see him, and he had brought his wife and her daughter and their son. They all had such a nice visit. You could see the joy in Cheyenne's eyes, and it was good for him.

Misty and Brent stuck around through the weekend and we made the most of our time together. We did some shopping, but just mostly visiting with each other. Riley was starting to say some different things and he so loved playing right in the middle of both of his brothers. He would have a fit if they tried to shut him out or ignore him. He could not tattle, but he could. It was funny.

Even though we'd just had Christmas, we went to the toy store one day, because they were having a great sale. We all loaded up and went over to the mall. Heather and Troy were there with us also, and we headed through the maze together with the three young ones. Riley was in the stroller and he was just leaned back like he knew what was going to happen. He had it all figured out. There were a few things that they did not get from anyone and we were at the perfect store, so yes we caved. They each got a little something. Cheyenne got a Star Wars action figure and Zachary got a pack of little cars and Riley got some of the little people he liked so well.

Riley was really starting to like playing with little toy people and he also loved anything with Scooby-Doo on it, about it or Scooby himself. Also, we had found that there were a few movies Riley would hold still for. They were *Bear and the Big Blue House*, *Stewart Little* and *Scooby-Doo, I love you*.

We got home from the mall and everyone was exhausted. The day just drifted by it seemed. Dinner was always fun with such a big crowd, and Riley loved to eat so it wasn't too hard to please him. He really loved his ice cream, but a lot of times it did not like him, so we had to be careful how much he would try to eat.

The time flew and it was time for them to leave and drive back to

Arkansas. I was tired but still did not like that they were leaving. It was just so difficult to say goodbye. I missed them so much when they were gone. I hated that they lived so far away from me. Yes, it was selfish, but I did not care.

CHAPTER SEVENTEEN

2004 CAME IN WITH A bang. Another new beginning. What would become of us all this New Year? I loved starting over, newness again. The anticipation is what was fun.

Misty and I both were with the same telephone company and they had just come out with a flat rate per month no matter how long you talked or where in the country you called. It was perfect and we were put on the plan almost simultaneously without knowing what we were doing. So we truly stayed in touch. We talked at least once a day if not more. Some say that is a little too much. I say "Ehhhhh!" I love talking to her about everything and she seems to love talking with me. It's like we are best friends and not mother-daughter. Having Riley in our lives has brought us closer in different and better ways. I don't know that everyone can understand. But maybe they don't have to, just accept how we cope and deal and relate with each other is all.

Misty had started doing some scrapbooking. She had discovered it was fun, relaxing and creative. She and her friend Dawn would go for hours at a time to make a page or two, but they were incredible. She made me a beautiful album for Christmas that is a true treasure. I told her she should do it for other people and make a little money for herself. She finally had an outlet that would take her in all different directions.

One day as I was shopping for fabric to make something else, I noticed a pattern for a scrapbooking apron. *Well,* I thought, *this would be a great present for Misty. I could make two, one for Misty and one for Dawn. I could get alternating fabrics and colors.* I immediately found fabric and bought the pattern and went to work. It took me two weeks to finish in my spare time, but they were finally done. So I boxed them up and mailed them out. I made two women very happy, which made my day. Dawn took a picture with her digital camera of the two of them and emailed it to me. What a great invention, digital cameras…every grandmother should have one.

Business had started to pick up some, so I was at least staying busier at work and having less time on my hands to worry or think. There is solace in staying busy and I really did try to stay busy. I coped better when I was keeping up with other things. The people in our office are terrific. We are all more of a family than at any other place I have worked or been a part of in the past. At any rate, it was not as easy to get away and travel as I had wanted. I had to plan and use more weekend time.

Heather and I decided we needed to go see them by the end of February, so I made reservations.

Meanwhile, my sister was getting married on Valentine's Day. It was great because I got to help her do some things in preparation, and our office threw her a surprise lingerie shower. What a hoot! My mom helped us deceive her and it was such fun decorating with red and white and the food, so much food, so much good food. It all was a great distraction.

February 14, 2004 and north Texas got about four inches of the most beautiful snow I have seen. I was up at eight a.m. and I called Marlene to see how she was holding up and I got hold of a panicked bride. She was worried about everything, which is totally normal, but she did not think her wedding would happen. I knew better, because I was not the bride-to-be. The snow was wet, the temperature was not that cold and it was melting on the roads as the morning wore on.

Her wedding turned out beautiful. She had a small audience, but we were the lucky ones that day. It was over before we knew it. Another V-Day with a twist.

Heather and I flew to Arkansas at the end of February. It was a chore getting everything together to go again. However, there was our Riley Joe at the airport. He ran for the two of us, such a cutie. Cheyenne was subdued but happy to see us. He loved his Aunt Heather. The ride back to the house was always a good time to catch up. We worked hard to keep Riley awake in the car. He loved to sing along with the radio and he really does act as though he is singing with passion, his face all scrunched up just goggling nonsense at us with such enthusiasm.

When we got to the house we just plopped down and started hashing out what we might do while we were there. At one point Misty started to get on to Cheyenne for interrupting and he talked back to her and they were on an ugly collision course. Well, that just did not set well with Riley. He went and tugged on her, looked up at her and started crying. She knew what was going on. He could not stand for there to be discord in his family. He would let you know in his own way that he did not tolerate it well…and that was the end of the argument.

That night we went to see that new movie together that was hyped everywhere, *The Passion of the Christ*. We all agreed that it was a profound movie and we were glad to see it together.

The next day, we were up early and on the road by nine. First stop of the day was for breakfast. Oh how Riley loved to eat, he would get so excited. He now had to sit in a chair. No high chair for that little man, he wanted to be included with everyone.

We got to the mall and all emotions broke loose. Cheyenne wanted everything there was to have and Riley was not very happy either and no one knew why. It appeared they were revolting against us. I took Riley out of his stroller and we went for our own little walk up and down the huge aisles. He would take off and I was right smack behind him keeping up and that was a feat in and of itself for Momo! But it made him laugh and giggle. Cheyenne came with me just to make sure all was well with our little adventure. He has such a big kind heart.

Our trip to the mall was soon over, but not soon enough as I ended up spending way too much. Oh well, I knew I couldn't take it with me. On our way home we sang to the radio, played patty-cake and itsy bitsy spider.

That evening was a little calmer with dinner and a movie. Riley loved to watch his movies in his room. It was a limited selection; however, he just loved it. If it wasn't Riley wanting my attention, it was Cheyenne wanting me to watch a movie with him. It was the most popular I had ever been!

CHAPTER EIGHTEEN

IT WAS TIME FOR SPRING break and the Hoofers, as we fondly referred to them, were coming to Texas for a visit. They would have all three boys with them. It would be an extended weekend but we could all go to Six Flags Over Texas one day and the other two days we would figure it out.

They came in on a Thursday and I raced home from work to greet them. I missed them all so much, I just could not hug and kiss enough. Heather and Troy came over and the party was complete. Riley immediately made a dash for the toys. Cheyenne and Zachary went out to the backyard to play. We ordered pizza and sat around and laughed and talked until it was time for bed.

The next day they decided to go to the Fort Worth Zoo. I went to work. At the end of the day we ended up at the house about the same time. They had a terrific time. Of course, if you have ever been to our zoo then you know how great it is. Riley was worn out. He had fallen asleep on the way home, and Misty got him into the bedroom before he woke up.

Saturday came and the boys were excited to go to Six Flags. Bob could not go as he had to be at work, so I rode with Misty and Brent, and then Heather and Troy met us at the park. We got there bright and early, but for some reason our Mr. Riley was not happy and when we stopped to get a group picture as you walk in, he was in his stroller and he would not lift his head for anybody. He was mad. So now we have this wonderful group picture and Riley has his head down—what a character.

We took turns swapping out the bigger boys and bigger rides for the younger rides with Riley. Oh, he did have fun. He would point and sign what he wanted, and he laughed on the rides. It was nonstop fun. We had to give up at about two in the afternoon. The day was warm and the adults were done!

They left the next morning before we even got up to get an early start. I was so sad all day I couldn't stand it. We did have a good visit and everyone enjoyed the time. One thing we have to try to keep in mind, at least with Riley, is that children with special needs are still children and should be treated as normally as possible.

It was routines again, waiting for the break and the time we would see each other again. We spoke every day on the phone, and Misty was telling me everything Riley was learning at home and at school. She had even gotten a book on sign language and was using it to teach him more signs. I was learning a few things along the way. I thought it was hard to learn but I wanted to try.

Cheyenne was struggling in school again as his medications did not seem to be working anymore. His ADHD had Misty and Brent at their wits' end with attitude and respect. He knew how he needed to act but for some reason he was not very enthusiastic about behaving that way. The doctors were trying some different meds. It was one of those see-and-wait situations. He was soon to turn eleven years old, and Misty did not know what to do for him that year.

It was decided that she would just have a family birthday that year and she would let him have his half brother from Fort Worth come up with his family. He was very happy over getting to see them.

We celebrated on a Saturday and the weather was beautiful. I was there. I had flown in the night before. Misty had a Sponge Bob Square Pants cake and theme. He had all his cousins and his family from Fort Worth and the place was packed. I had bought him rollerblades and he was happy. Riley and Zachary were there and there were so many kids, the adults were very outnumbered. Riley was so busy with his playing he was just fun to watch, going from person to person, activity to activity. He did not stop until almost everyone was gone and we found him on the floor of the living room sound asleep, I swear. He was even snoring. The rest of us decided to watch *Spy Kids 3* with the 3-D glasses. I enjoyed that movie more than I expected.

The next day I had to leave and it was a long lonely drive to the airport. Riley was asleep when I got out of the car. So I kissed him on the cheek and told them to go home, I would call later. The flight home, although less than an hour, was long and then I had to deal with a parking garage under construction when I got home.

I cannot believe that they get away with charging you to park in a garage you cannot find your way around in, and you feel scared to death walking around in it. But they do and no one cares until something terrible happens to some unknowing patron. Oh well, enough of that. I got home late that night and just fell into bed exhausted.

CHAPTER NINETEEN

TWO MONTHS PASSED AND I could not stand it anymore. I told Heather, "We have to go see them, it has been way too long. Maybe you can drive and Troy and Bob can go with us?"

She agreed, so off we went with her, Troy and I. Bob had to work the weekend. We left after work on a Friday and it was a nightmare getting out of Dallas. To make matters worse it was raining when we left, so traffic was in slow motion. It took us longer to get there than it had ever taken before. We got there about midnight. Misty was up waiting on us and everyone else was asleep. We looked in on Riley. He was so cute asleep with his dad, and we went to bed.

The next morning we were greeted with giggles and googles. It was so great. We tickled and ran and tickled and ran for at least an hour. I wore him out good, then gave him his bath. He loved his bath. He played, I splashed, he swam, I rinsed him, he drank the water, I chastised him, and he ignored me.

An hour later we were dressed and eating the best homemade breakfast ever. Dawn and Rachel showed up and it was really festive as I had bought the cutest Barbie swimsuit with a pink grass skirt and sunglasses to match...talk about cute, she loved it. Of course I had brought something for Riley and Cheyenne. Heather had gotten a swimsuit for Riley that was as cute as it could be also.

After breakfast, you guessed it, we were off to the mall. We shopped a long while, mostly to kill time as we were going to meet Brent's sister and her boyfriend for dinner at a restaurant on the wharf. But we did find a few treasures we could not do without. Riley and I went up and down the big corridors in the mall to get him out of his stroller. He loved to run away from me, he thought it was funny. Yes, we wore each other out, mostly me.

Dinner was nice. It was on the water and the food was good. Brent's sister looked good and we all had a nice visit. Riley got his food first. Misty always tried to get him something first to prevent any anxious hungry moments. It worked pretty well that way, she had a good plan. The restaurant had a huge fish tank that Riley was just enamored with; it was beautiful. There were a lot of different fish in the tank it was so large.

After dinner we were on our way. It was late and the boys were tired. Riley was asleep in five minutes, Cheyenne ten. Heather, Troy, Brent, Misty and I visited the rest of the way home. It was a good time. When we were home, we ended up calling it a night.

The next morning was a rush to shower, pack and eat. By time we were all ready it was noon. It was time to go. It was so hard to say goodbye. When it came time to kiss Riley goodbye, he started crying. When we got in the car to leave he reached for me and had real tears. I could not believe it. He really realized I was leaving and he did not want me to go. He knew me…he loved me…oh my! That was it, that was where I wanted us to be. Now I knew it was all worth the struggle. Riley knew I was his momo!

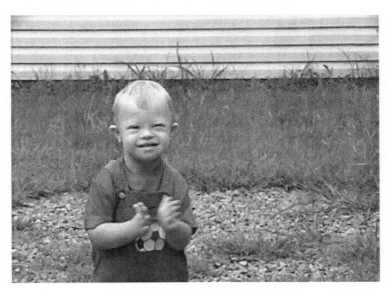